This book was inspired by Mary "May" Mohan and is dedicated in her memory and honor.

Table of Contents

Introduction

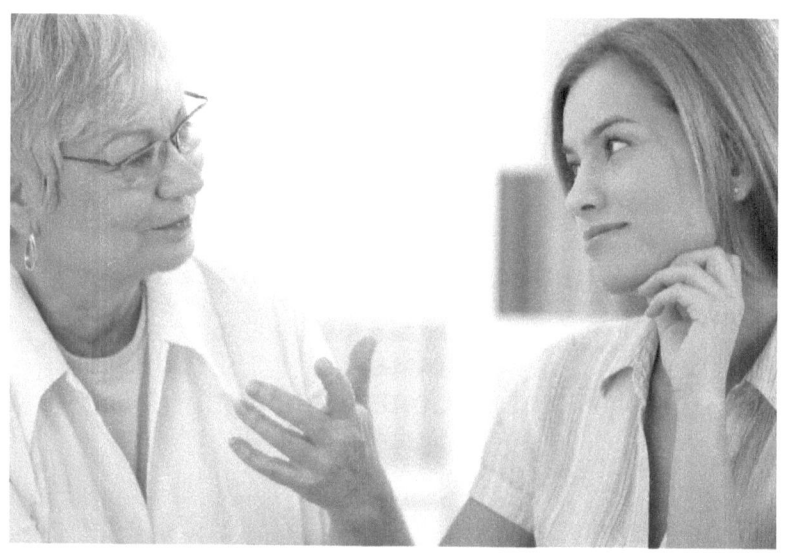

Everyone knows people with hearing loss, but few people know how to effectively communicate with them. Difficulties arise when a person with normal hearing makes assumptions about what may be helpful to a person with a hearing loss. Therefore, we have written this practical guide for anyone interested in how to talk to people with hearing loss (especially family, friends and the general public).

The purpose of this book is to tell you what people with hearing loss find useful from their communication partners, so that you can be a better communicator. Sometimes, you might find that people with hearing loss shut down when you try to talk to them, or they might react badly to your efforts to communicate. To avoid this, it helps to understand how people with hearing loss actually hear. Because we often make wrong assumptions about how they hear, we start by dispelling myths and answering common questions. Then we explain how you can communicate most effectively.

The information in this book is based on solid science and experience. Because not everyone is interested in the science of hearing-loss communication, we leave out research studies and the scientific jargon. We tell you what to do in plain language. If you want more scientific data, there are many other places to find it.

Before we begin, we would like to share a story about the woman who was the inspiration for this book.

A True Story

Mary "May" Mohan was the daughter of immigrants and lived the American Dream with persistence, kindness, and humility. She was hardworking and dedicated to her loved-ones, which included her family, neighbors, wider community, and animals.

May Mohan was a natural teacher; she enjoyed solving problems and sharing what she discovered. She delighted in communicating with children, and she always seemed to have a flock of them around her tiny summer cottage on the edge of a forest with tall pine trees.

Because of her hearing loss, May taught the children how to communicate with her. When a little girl started talking with her hands in front of her mouth, May would gently move her arm away and say, "I need to see your sweet face to be able to hear you." The child may not have understood why, but she smiled and complied. (Most adults did not speak so gently to children and most children seemed to appreciate the way she talked to them.)

Sometimes, May would say things that sounded a bit crazy until she explained. As she became older and her vision started to become worse, she made the observation, "I hear better with my glasses on." Puzzled looks invited her to explain, "There are sounds I cannot hear, but I can see them when I look at your faces." (She discovered some of the things that you will learn in this book.)

If you were invited into May's house, you were expected to be polite. Mid-afternoons she would serve tea, lemonade, and sometimes something delicious! The television was turned off during her afternoon teas. Tea time was for talking, not for watching the television.

In May's house, people were encouraged to do one thing at a time and do it well. When one person talked, the others would listen. Interrupting was impolite. Each person would be given time to talk, as May guided the always interesting and often funny conversation.

While never preaching, May was frequently teaching communication skills through her good example. No one could listen to children like May and the children loved her for the gift of attention she gave them!

May taught manners, but she also ensured that she could understand the children. By having the rule that they took turns speaking, she could follow the conversation. By sitting in a circle, she could see the face of each guest. She was a communication specialist without any formal training!

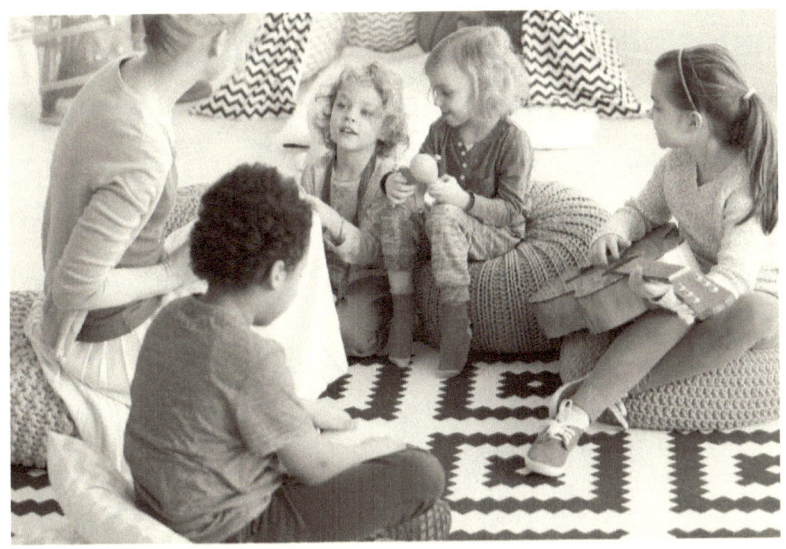

May Mohan firmly believed in collective action among like-minded human beings to improve society. She believed that local action could solve many problems. May and her sister cooked meals for neighbors who could not cook, and she organized a delivery system using kids on bikes or "runners" on foot.

The authors believe that May would approve of this book. It came about through the inspiration and urging of many people to provide information on better communication strategies. Simply put: How to Talk to People with Hearing Loss. Therefore, this book was inspired by Mary "May" Mohan and is dedicated in her memory and honor.

Book Outline

This book covers the most common problems associated with communication breakdowns. Its focus is short and sharp: what you can do to help.

In Chapter 1, we consider myths about hearing loss and tell you the truth about the way people with hearing loss hear, based on scientific research. In Chapter 2, we discuss issues related to avoiding conflicts caused by misconceptions of hearing loss.

In Chapter 3, we tell you what people with hearing loss say really helps them better communicate and examine why it helps. Because having the knowledge of what is important does not ensure that we can do it, we make suggestions for actions that are helpful for improving communication. Once you are aware of what to do, it requires work to take new actions.

New habits can be hard to learn. So, Chapter 4 emphasizes the importance of practice, and gives you tips on developing better communication habits.

We hope you find this guide helpful! If there is some information that you want included in future editions of this book or if you have a story to tell, let us know. We would love to hear from you at

TalkToPeopleWithHearingLoss@gmail.com

This guide should take less than an hour to read. After that, you'll be able to practice on your own. Let's get started!

Chapter One

Two Major Myths About Hearing Loss

We have noticed two very common misconceptions about hearing loss that often cause communication problems. Before we go any further, let's bust these myths.

Myth One

People with hearing loss do not notice or "hear" sounds unless you shout at them.

Family members are surprised when a grandparent with hearing loss complains about a teenager's loud music. Neighbors are often puzzled when a person with hearing loss complains about neighborhood noise. They wonder, how does this happen when the person has such difficulty hearing?

People with hearing loss can hear loud sounds and they may also hear some softer sounds. A person with hearing loss can be bothered by construction noise and loud music in the next apartment. This is because they still can hear low-pitched sounds, like the thumps of

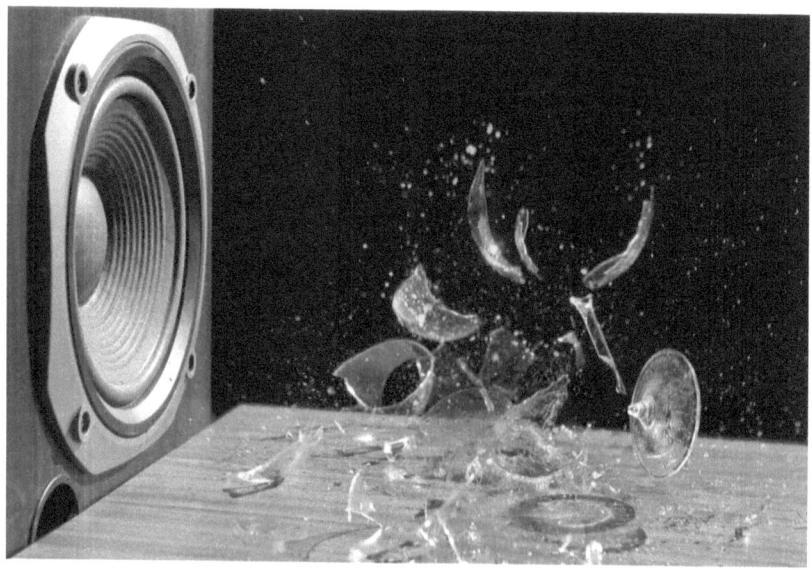

construction noise or the bass sounds of loud music.

Some people with hearing loss may even hear loud sounds louder than the average person without hearing loss. This is called "hyperacusis" and loud sounds can be so bothersome that they cannot enjoy the loud parts of movies in neighborhood theaters.

Myth Two

Hearing aids correct hearing to normal or near normal, much like eyeglasses. If a person with hearing loss just wore their hearing aids, all their communication problems would be solved.

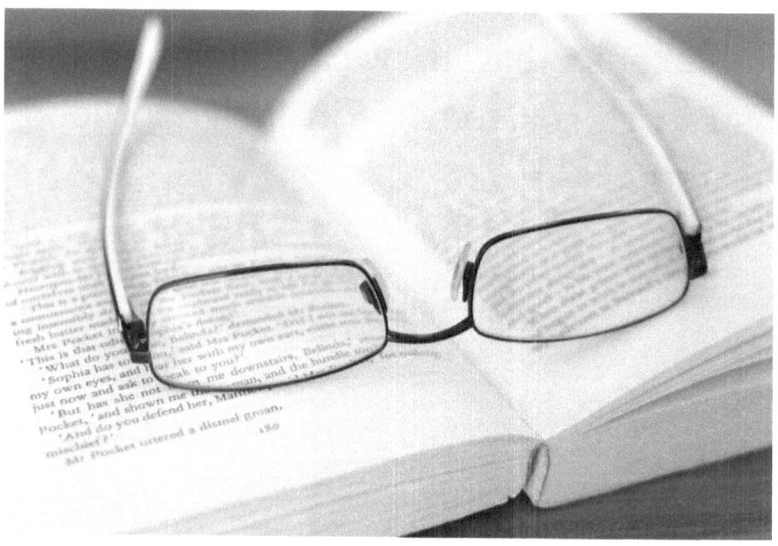

Correcting the most common forms of visual problems (nearsightedness and farsightedness) is simply a problem of bending the light with lenses to correct the eye shape, which makes it focus correctly. The problem of hearing loss is more complex.

Hearing loss can be a problem of transmission in the ear ("conductive loss") or processing in the nerves to the brain ("sensorineural loss") or both. Conductive hearing loss could be caused by problems such as fluid in the ear or a wax blockage. Sensorineural hearing loss (including distortion, lack of clarity, and/or volume difficulties) could be caused by damage due to loud sound exposure or hereditary factors. Typically, with age-related hearing loss, the problem with processing involves communicating sound to the brain and making sense of it. This problem makes it more difficult to differentiate important sounds from background noise. People with hearing loss can often detect sounds, but these sounds blend more easily with the background, making words harder to understand.

The processing can be damaged in various ways that scientists are still only beginning to understand. There are large differences among people with hearing losses in their abilities to process information. All hearing losses are not the same. If hearing loss is only a simple transmission problem, like visual acuity loss, a simple hearing aid that amplifies sounds could return hearing to normal or near normal. People with complex sensorineural hearing losses may need more sophisticated hearing aids.

Hearing-aid innovations are helpful, but no hearing-aid available today can entirely compensate for most types of hearing loss. No one has the ability yet to replace the intricate machinery of the ear or the nerves themselves. In complex listening environments (such as loud restaurants or parties) and under difficult listening situations (such as with non-native speakers and fast talkers), people with age-related hearing loss have difficulty hearing even when they use their hearing aids.

Chapter Two
Five Most Common Questions Answered

Understanding what people with hearing loss think can help you avoid conflicts. If we understand how the person with hearing loss is hearing, we gain insight into what they say and what they do.

Things that some people with hearing losses may say can start an argument, such as "Don't shout, I can hear you." or "Don't mumble." Let's try to answer some of the questions we received from family members.

Why do they tell you not to shout when they barely can hear?

This is a topic that we know a lot about because we have done the research! Not all people with hearing loss hear sounds in the same way. In fact, there can be large differences in the way two people hear a sound. If the two people are sitting in the same car and an ambulance with a siren passes them, the siren may sound very loud to one person and soft to the other.

Many people with hearing loss cannot hear soft sounds, but they can of course hear loud sounds. When they do hear loud sounds, they can sound about as loud as they do for people without a hearing loss. This leads to many misunderstandings in countless families. This is an example of what happens: a girl is asked to go to another room and tell her grandfather, who has a hearing loss, something. She enters the room and he doesn't notice her. She says, "Grandfather" and he does not hear her. She raises her voice a little and repeats, "Grandfather" and he still does not hear her. She then makes her voice very loud, "GRANDFATHER" and he hears her for the first time with her loud voice. The grandfather tells her in a stern voice, "Don't shout! I can hear you!" The girl is upset and wonders why he tells her not to shout when he can barely hear.

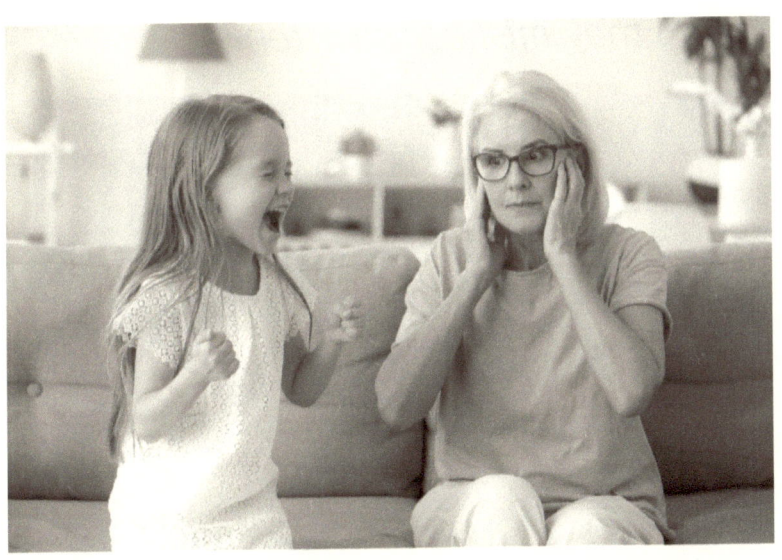

We have taught many children how to talk to people with hearing losses using the 10 tips given in Chapter 3. Most children understand that a person cannot hear soft sounds, but can hear loud sounds. They just need to know what to do; most children are very happy to be helpful. These polite behaviors are easy for very young children to grasp when motivated by a loving grandparent. After all, most of these actions are simple civility.

Why do they mishear so often?

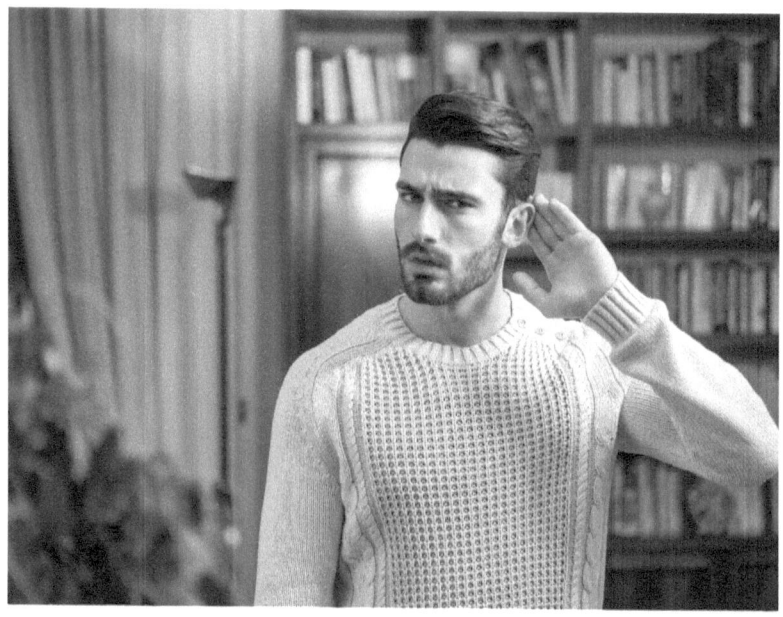

Having sounds loud enough, but not too loud, is not the only problem experienced by people with hearing losses. Most people also have varying amounts of difficulty hearing quick changes in speech over time. They may have difficulty following the pace of friendly conversations (about 110-150 words per minute), and are entirely lost trying to follow the pace of professional speakers (about 145-160 words per minute). Little wonder why they have no chance of following the medication warnings at the end of television commercials!

Sounds that are difficult to hear and fast speech cause them to understand only part of what is said. When this happens, the brain works to make sense of the available information and they mishear. Hearing words incorrectly ("mishearing") can happen in two ways:

1. What they hear makes sense to them and sounds logical, like the woman who heard on the radio about a program for weight loss that "used psychology and small bowls" only to discover later that it "used psychology and small goals"!

2. They are aware that they did not hear correctly and they guess. Sometimes they guess right; sometimes they guess wrong. When they guess incorrectly and respond to what they thought was said, their comment does not make sense.

Because mishearing is so common, it is important for the person with hearing loss to have another person accompany them to medical and legal appointments, or anywhere professional jargon is used. Professional jargon is especially susceptible to mishearing. One patient was told that he had "Sickle Cell anemia" and he heard it as "sick-as-hell anemia"! This example is funny, but it can be very serious when a patient mishears or does not understand the doctor.

Hearing loss can be incorrectly diagnosed as cognitive problems when the patient mishears and responds strangely or does not understand and asks no questions. It could be important to ask the patient to repeat what the doctor said to ensure that the patient understood.

Why don't they get a hearing aid?

From the time older adults have a hearing loss, they typically wait 10 to 15 years before they try a hearing aid for the first time. The cost of hearing aids can be a reason not to buy one, but there are also other reasons.

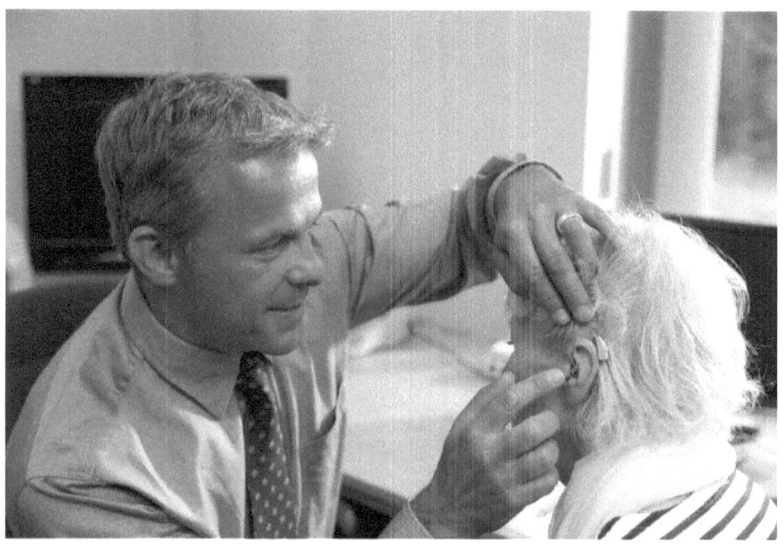

It takes time and they need to get to the point that they are missing too much and they want to do something about it. For one person, it could be missing the sounds of a loved-one's voice, such as a grandchild. For another, it may be that they are not getting the jokes and they realize that their friends are getting tired of repeating the jokes to them.

If a person is not ready to use a hearing aid, you really cannot make them. Many well-meaning family members have taken a person to buy a hearing aid before the person is ready. It needs to be the person's decision, not yours. Of course, you can support them, but you cannot decide for them.

This is why giving a hearing-aid as a birthday or holiday present is a bad idea. Unless a person asks for a hearing aid (just like a diet book, or a clutter guide), don't gift it!

Why don't they use a hearing aid once they have bought one?

After not hearing sounds for years, when a person puts on a hearing aid for the first time, they are bombarded by sounds. One man told his wife that the toilet flushing sounded like Niagara Falls!

It takes time and adjustment to get used to hearing aids. If they need help after the hearing-aid trial period has lapsed, they may think that it is their fault. After all

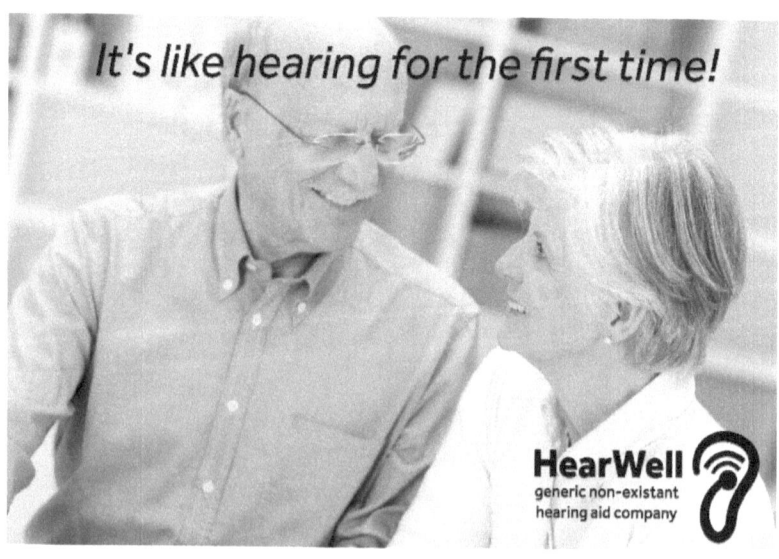

It's like hearing for the first time!

HearWell
generic non-existant
hearing aid company

the glossy ads and commercials with smiling people using hearing aids, they expect that their hearing will be fully restored and that this will happen without effort on their part. They feel that it is their fault when they have problems adjusting to their new hearing aids. Shame breeds silence and many are unlikely to ask for help. They may also feel guilty after spending all that money for hearing aids and then not using them.

Working out these issues is not easy. It takes time and effort, and expectations need to be realistic. Hearing aids work best in quiet environments by making soft sounds easier to hear. This reduces the listener's stress and tiredness caused by straining to hear. There are many listening situations in which hearing aids provide clear benefit and their owners are very happy with them.

There are other situations in which hearing aids provide only limited benefit. Background noise is a big problem. Although the technology associated with hearing aids has improved over the years, there is no hearing aid that can restore hearing back to pre-hearing-loss days. Unrealistic expectations of what hearing aids can do may cause people to be so disappointed that they give up trying to use them.

Why do they think that people mumble?

Most people with age-related hearing loss do not hear high-pitched sounds as well as they hear low-pitched sounds. Without hearing the high-pitched sounds, it sounds like people mumble or their voices are muffled. (To give you a rough idea of what speech may sound like to them, find a willing friend and ask them to speak to you with a bucket over their head. The bucket will block some of the high-pitched sounds and allow the low-

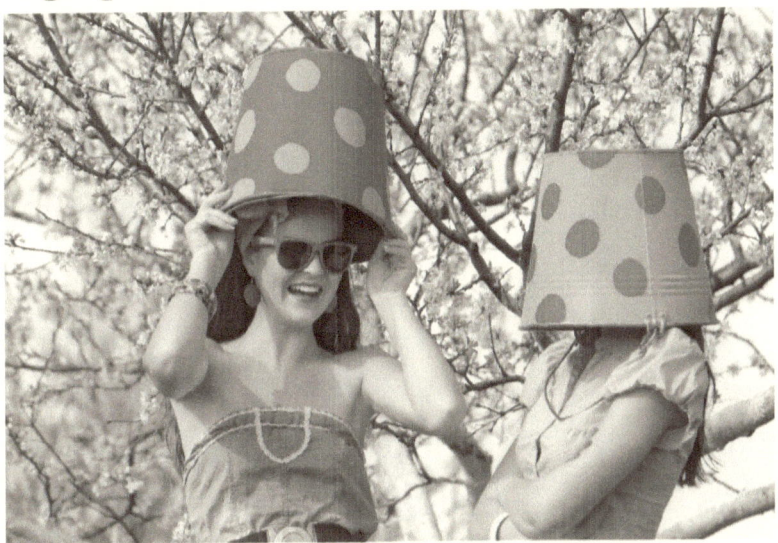

pitched sounds to arrive at your ears. You can also do this digitally, but a bucket or cardboard box might be quicker and more fun!)

When people with hearing loss are bothered by apparent mumbling, they usually complain to their friends of the same age. If they are of an older generation, at least one of their peers will hear the same way and agree with them. They confirm one another's belief that the problem is not their hearing; it is caused by the speaker's lack of articulation skills. They agree, "Elocution used to be taught in schools, but it has fallen out of the curriculum. That is why young people mumble!"

Many people are surprised to learn that nearly 25 percent of people aged 65 to 74 years have disabling hearing loss. In people over 75 years, over half of their peers will have debilitating hearing loss. (These statistics are published by the National Institutes of Health, Department of Health and Human Services; NIH-NIDCD website 2019).

If you are accused of mumbling or told to speak clearly, try to understand that this is how they hear, and they believe that they are correct. People's perceptions are real to them and it could take a lot of time to convince them otherwise. It may be easier to check that you are using the 10 tips in Chapter 3, which will give them the best chance of understanding your speech.

Chapter Three
Ten Tips for Effective Communication

To answer the question of what helps people with hearing loss, we asked different groups of older people in several countries and different places throughout the United States. This is what they said summarized into ten tips:

1. Get my attention before you start speaking to me.

2. Speak slowly and clearly. A moderate pace works best.

3. Look at me, take your hands away from your mouth, and don't exaggerate your pronunciation.

4. Don't raise your voice too loud; moderately loud is best.

5. If you are going to change the topic, tell me.

6. If I do not hear you the first time, repeat with different words. Don't say the same word I did not hear over and over again.

7. Try to limit or avoid background noise. I do not hear well in noisy environments.

8. Talk to me on the side of my better ear.

9. Gestures help me, but don't be too extreme.

10. Hearing under adverse conditions can be exhausting. Sometimes, I need a break.

These tips agree with what healthcare professionals tell us and are consistent with data from research experiments. We know this because we have done research ourselves and evaluated many research experiments. More importantly, we have discussed the issues related to hearing loss with many people who actually live with hearing loss. We know these tips work.

Now that we know what helps, let's examine one tip at a time to expand on what you could do to be helpful and why it works.

Tip One

"Get my attention before you start speaking to me."

It is important to get the person's attention so that they do not miss the first part of your sentence. This gives you the best chance of having your message received correctly the first time. If they do not hear you the first time, you will need to repeat or say it using different words. It not only takes more time, but it may get the conversation off to an unpleasant start.

What is a good way to get someone's attention? Enter their line of vision at a moderately slow pace. Be careful not to move too quickly. They may not hear you walking toward them, and you don't want to startle them.

Position yourself so that you are close enough that they can comfortably see

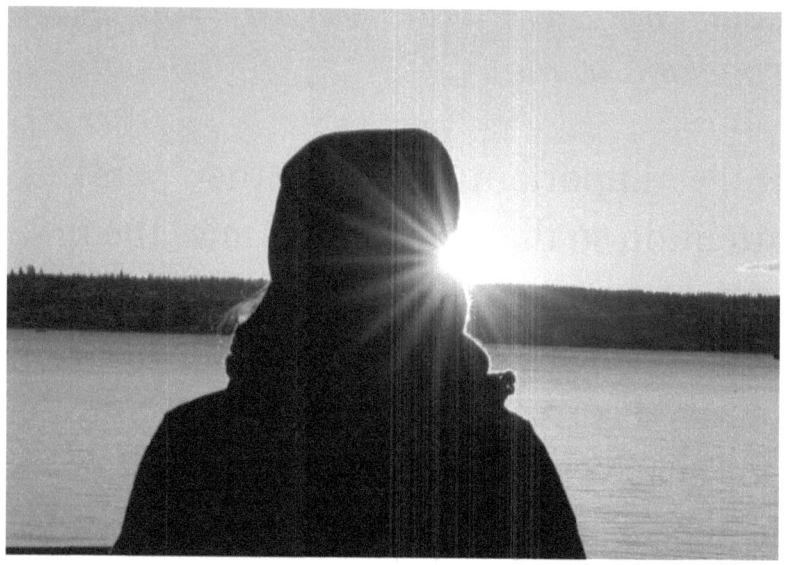

your mouth and your facial expressions. Be careful about lighting; if the sun or a bright light is behind you, they may not be able to see you. Next, look at them to signal that you are about to speak.

Use their name to let them know you will be talking to them. The sound of a person's name signals them to pay attention. Because listening requires effort for people with hearing loss, they have a tendency to tune-out when they do not need to listen. Using their name cuts through their attention filter and some of the background noise. It also signals to them to look at you. Now that you have prepared them to receive your message, start speaking.

In summary: Enter their line of vision so that they can clearly and comfortably see you. Use their name. Wait for them to look at you. Begin speaking.

Tip Two

"Speak slowly and clearly. A moderate pace works best."

It is best to keep a moderate pace. Talking too fast or too slow is not effective. If you talk too fast, the person will not be able to process your speech that quickly. If you talk too slowly, you will sound strange and the person might forget what you said at the beginning. Moderate pace with natural sounding speech works best.

Pausing between thoughts can be helpful. It gives the listener time to process what you said and question you if they need clarification. Long pauses can be effective in initiating a new topic.

If your accent or dialect is different from that of the listener, a little more time to process your message can be very beneficial. It takes time for our brains to get used to accents, dialects, and languages that are other than our first language.

In summary: Speak clearly at a moderate pace with pauses between thoughts.

Tip Three

"Look at me, take your hands away from your mouth, and don't exaggerate your pronunciation."

Many people have learned to use visual information from the mouth and facial expressions along with the sounds they receive to understand speech. The words "bother" and "father" sound very similar to people with age-related hearing loss, but they look different when they are being said. The lips come together for "bother" to make a puff of air to start the word; the air coming through the mouth is continuous at the start of "father."

Using these cues to understand speech is called "speechreading." It used to be called "lip reading," but we now know that we use more than information from the lips. Facial expressions also help.

Although there are excellent speechreading courses, some people learn to speech read on their own without formal training. If you met a friend, who you had not seen in awhile, and said, "Hello! How are you?" without making any sound (just moving your mouth while maintaining the right facial expression), it is likely that your friend could guess what you said. Whether a person has had formal training speechreading or not, be sure that they can see your face.

Although many words can be speechread, others cannot. If you go to the mirror and say "mom, bomb," in a natural manner and speed, they look the same on your lips. Speechreading can be helpful, but do not expect that a speechreader can understand all speech 100% of the time using speechreading alone.

Many people exaggerate their pronunciation because they think it will make them easier to understand, but it can actually make it worse. Exaggerated pronunciation changes speechreading cues and may bring unwanted attention from others who can see you. Speak naturally. Whatever you do, try not to bring attention to the person with hearing loss. Most people feel uncomfortable with actions that draw attention when they are in public.

If you are eating while talking, make sure that you swallow the food in your mouth before you start to talk. Holding food in your mouth while talking will change the speechreading cues. Your parents were right, don't talk with your mouth full!

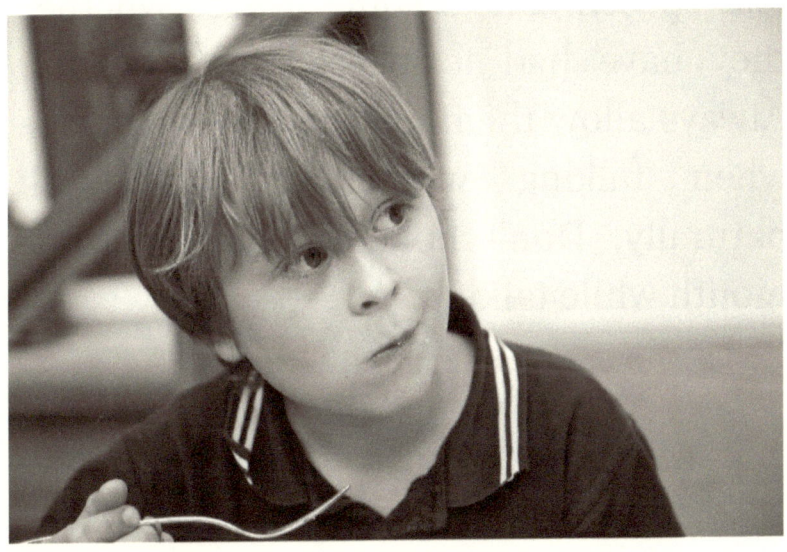

Perhaps these final suggestions are not needed, but people frequently do them without thinking. Don't talk in the dark; good lighting is important. Don't talk when sitting beside someone in a movie theater; they probably will not understand you. Don't talk from the other room unless the listener has superpowers and can see through walls!

In summary: Most people with hearing loss speechread to some degree whether they have had formal training or not. Always allow them to see your entire face when talking with them and talk naturally. Don't hold anything in your mouth while talking.

Tip Four

"Don't raise your voice too loud; moderately loud is best."

Most people with age-related hearing loss cannot hear soft sounds, but they do hear loud sounds. In fact, many people with hearing loss are especially bothered by loud sounds.

Shouting never works. It annoys people. Even if a shout is heard softly or quietly, it still sounds like a shout. The same is true of whispers. When whispers are recorded and played back at various sound levels, they can be identified as whispers whether they are heard soft or loud. Even when very loud, a whisper sounds better than a shout, because of the emotional response we have when someone is shouting at us.

No one likes to be shouted at. It can be difficult to speak at the right volume, but even young children can learn to do it.

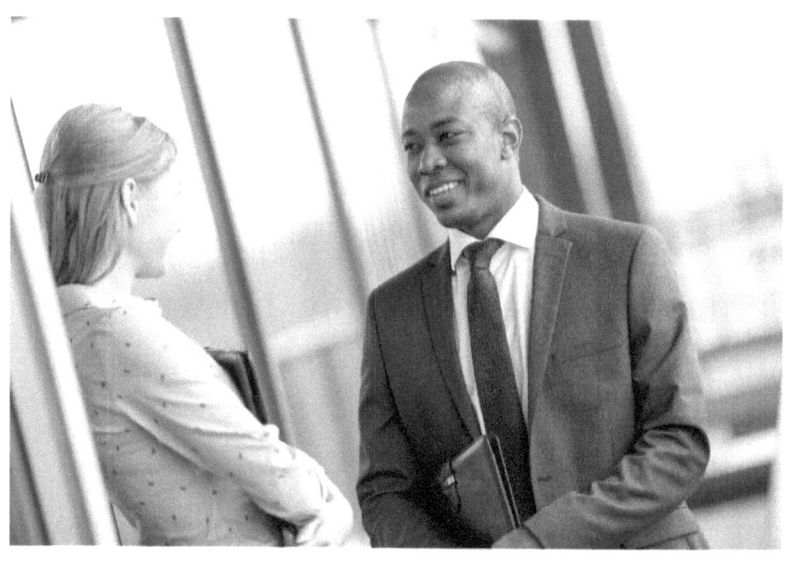

Speak at a moderate loudness if a person is wearing hearing aids. This should work if the hearing aids are working properly. If a person does not have hearing aids, you may have to raise your voice a bit. You may also move closer to your listener, which is another way of increasing the loudness of your voice.

If you move closer to the listener to make your voice louder, watch for body language. Each person has a zone of intimate space around them. Getting too close may make them feel uncomfortable, or may signal them that you wish to become sexually intimate. Be careful and move with caution!

In summary: Never shout. Instead, speak moderately loud. Sometimes it can help to move closer, but not uncomfortably close.

Tip Five

"If you are going to change the topic, tell me. Context helps me."

Context helps all of us understand when we are in challenging listening conditions. We predict what comes next based on what has been heard. It is very difficult for some people to follow a conversation when the flow jumps around from topic to topic.

One member of a conversation group became frustrated with a friend who kept jumping from topic to topic. There seemed to be no logical progression of ideas. He found himself exerting increasing effort to understand his friend. Despite his effort, he could not keep up with the conversation. Eventually, he laughed and told his friend, "Give me a turn signal!"

There are ways to introduce a new topic and give someone a signal that the topic of conversation is turning. You could say, "Now, I would like to talk with you about ..." or "On another topic, ..." There are many things you could say. Find one that feels natural to you.

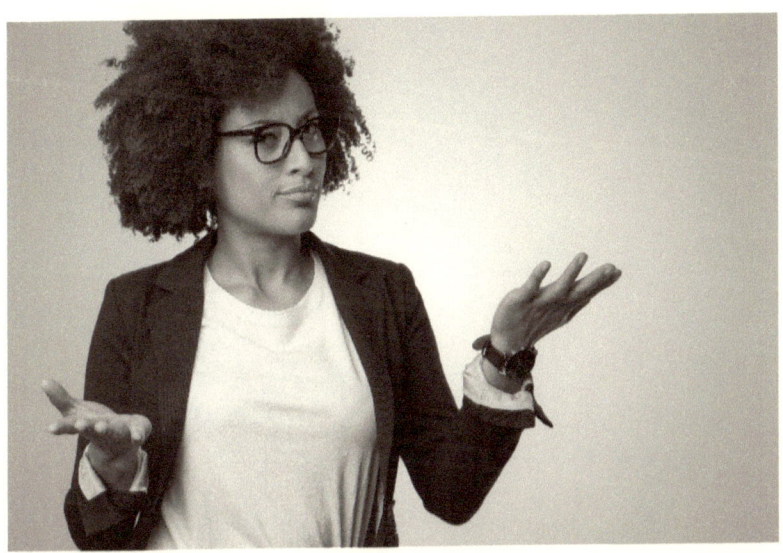

If you know a person well, you could have some signal like a gesture that feels natural. When talking in a group, you could repeat a few words to indicate a change of topic if you think that someone in the group needs a "turn signal."

In summary: Avoid changing topics without giving notice. Instead, clearly introduce new topics with common phrases or gestures.

Tip Six

"If I do not hear you the first time, repeat with different words."

Some words are more difficult to hear than other words. When a person with hearing loss misses a word, they often ask the speaker to repeat what they said. Most people will repeat the word that the person did not hear the first time.

If the listener does not hear the word again, some people continue to say the same word. Each time the word gets a little louder. This situation is extremely annoying to both the speaker and the listener.

If a person does not hear a word, it may be because the sound of that word might be especially difficult for them to process, and they do not have enough context to help them piece together the meaning. Saying the same thing with different words is a better strategy; it gives them another way to understand the message. If the word is an object and you both can see it, point or gesture. Writing or texting the word can be useful.

Even if you are having difficulty getting them to understand what you are saying, never give up and say, "Never mind." You may think that what you have to say may not be that important, and you may be right. But, the person with hearing loss wants to know what you said and is likely to feel left out. If you are having difficulty getting someone to understand, or you need to finish the conversation, it is better to say, "I'll tell you later." If you say this, remember to tell them later or they will not believe you the next time.

The I'll-tell-you-later response can work well when the conditions for communication are bad or when you need time to think of another way to say it with different words. Let's face it; sometimes it is exhausting to think of new ways to explain something. You may need a break to rest up.

In summary: If a person with hearing loss does not hear you the first or second time, pause and try a different way to communicate. Use other words, point, or write. Never resort to saying, "Never mind."

Tip Seven

"Try to limit or avoid background noise. I do not hear well in noisy environments."

It is difficult for people without hearing loss to understand the impact of background noise on a person with age-related hearing loss. This is because they hear differently. People without hearing loss efficiently filter out unwanted noise, except when in the most extreme noise environments. People with hearing loss experience varying amounts of difficulty doing the same thing.

Every time we listen, unless we are in a sound-isolating chamber, we hear the sounds we want to hear mixed with sounds that we do not want to hear. The sounds we do not want to hear are called "background noise."

We usually get used to it and "tune out" low-level background noises, such as the hum of a refrigerator or ventilation system fans; we don't even notice them. If we listen to the ventilation system, we actually can hear it go on and off, but we have to pay attention to hear it because we are so good at tuning out low-level continuous sounds. We can also tune out most other background noises, except when it gets very loud and/or really bothers us, like when a buzzing insect flies by.

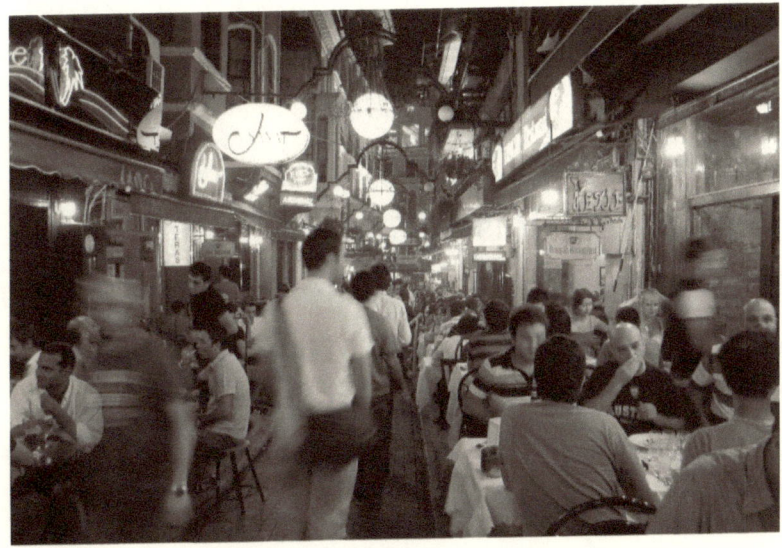

People with hearing loss have difficulty separating out unwanted sounds. Most very low-level sounds are usually not a problem because they are not heard. Moderate and loud sounds that mix with speech can be a big problem. Noisy restaurants are always a problem, although there are ways to minimize the problem. You could go at a less crowded time, or ask for a quiet table away from the kitchen and the bar. If that doesn't work, vote with your feet and go to another restaurant with better acoustics. You can look for reviews of quiet restaurants and even rate them yourself.

At home, you have more control of background noise. You can simply turn off the television or radio. If the person with hearing loss is watching television and you need to speak to them, ask them to put the television on pause or mute. If noise is coming from the hall, you can shut the door.

A home has many other things that make background sounds. Don't talk while washing dishes in the kitchen sink, using a food processor, or any other appliance that makes noise. Seek ways to reduce background noise or find a quiet place to talk. There are ways to quiet your home that are relatively inexpensive.

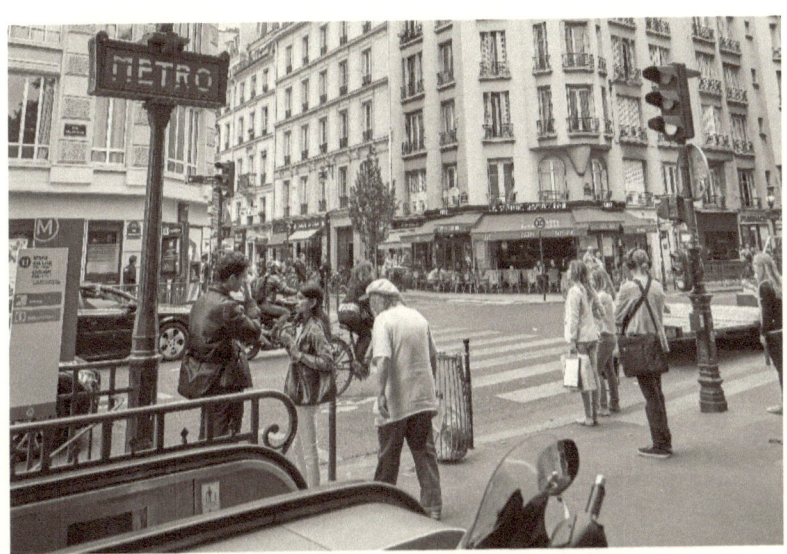

Outside the home, you have less control of noise. It is usually best not to try to talk while walking outside on a noisy street or in a public restroom, which can be an acoustic nightmare.

Flushing toilets, sinks with rushing water, and hand blow dryers make very loud and unpleasant noise that is made worse by the tiled walls and floor (hard surfaces like this can create an echo and make changes to the sound). In these kinds of environments, it is best to not even try to communicate until you are out of them.

In summary: Seek ways to limit background noise or wait until you are in a better environment to communicate.

Tip Eight

"Talk to me on the side of my better ear."

Although age-related hearing loss affects both ears, some people with hearing loss have a preferred listening ear. If they do, you have a better chance of getting your message through their preferred ear if you can position yourself on the correct side. If they are unsure of which ear is best, just ask them which ear they use to

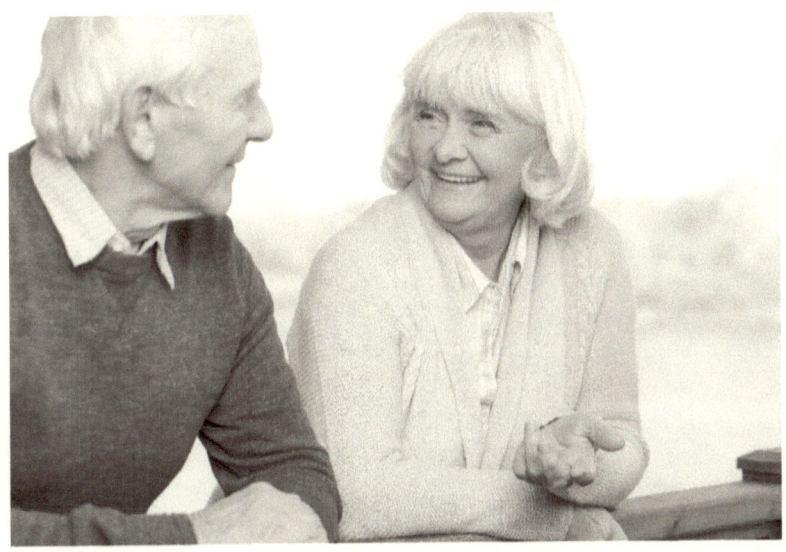

listen to the phone. If there is a difference between the ears, that will be the better ear.

For those people with better hearing in one ear, positioning yourself on the side of their better ear can make a big difference. When hosting guests, you can make communication easier with clever seating arrangements.

In summary: Identify their preferred ear and adapt accordingly.

Tip Nine

"Gestures help me, but don't be too extreme."

Relevant gestures, such as pointing to the object you refer to, can be very helpful, but be careful how you use them. Large and/or exaggerated hand movements can attract attention from across a room.

Never draw attention to yourself or the person that you are trying to help. Most people do not want attention drawn to their hearing loss. Of course, gestures are different from Sign Language. Sign Language is an accepted way to communicate in public spaces. Exaggerated or bizarre gestures will draw attention, especially from those who understand Sign Language!

In summary: Gestures can be useful, but
be subtle.

Tip Ten

"Hearing under adverse conditions can be exhausting. Sometimes, I need a break."

If you have something that takes time to say, break it up with pauses. Give the listener a chance to ask a question if something is unclear, or just rest a little. People with hearing loss need to work harder to piece together what they have difficulty hearing. Sometimes they need a rest.

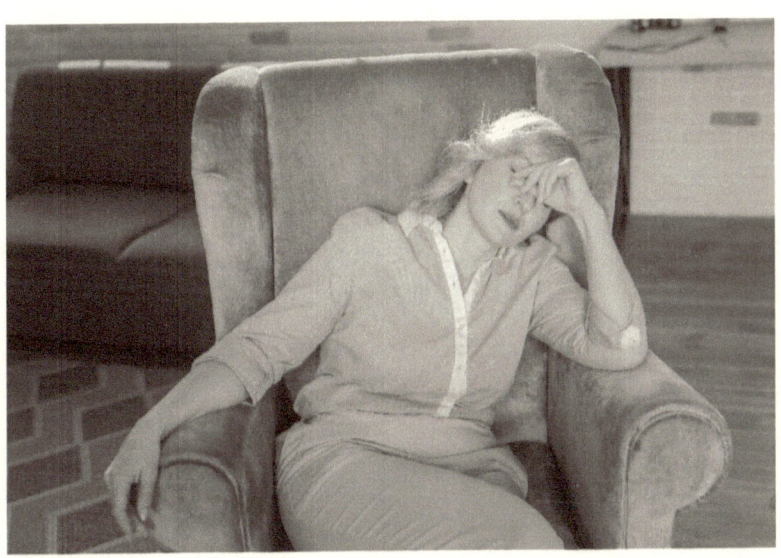

In summary: Make pauses in your speech to allow them to clarify and rest.

Chapter Four
Knowing is Not Enough

Perhaps you are familiar with the phrase "knowing is not doing"? Once we have firmly established a habit, information alone is not enough to change that habit. Our personal communication skills are such that gaining new patterns of behavior require practice.

Expect that you will make mistakes. None of us who have changed our behaviors have done it without making mistakes. You may start talking without getting the person's attention. It happens. Just self-correct and keep trying. To use a sports metaphor: if your game is not going well, your inner coach can suggest adjustments at half-time!

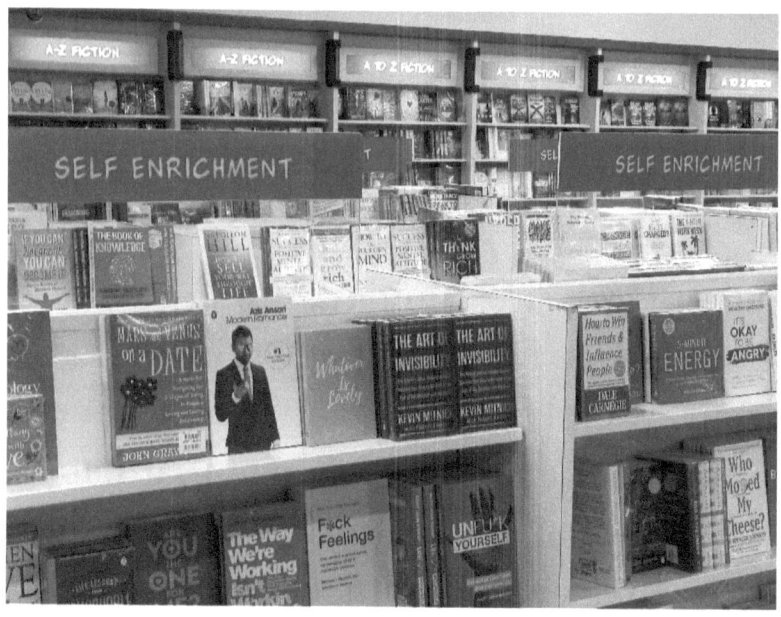

Habits are hard to change, even when people are highly motivated. Just think of a simple habit of eating snacks while watching television or getting rid of clutter in your house or office. If you already have the established habits of eating in front of the television, it is very difficult to stop. Even if you take the snacks off the coffee table, you may find yourself mindlessly going into the kitchen. Likewise, if you have established the habits of a clutter bug, simply reading good information rarely helps. Even if one does a clean-up and puts things in order, the clutter returns if certain behaviors are not changed.

The reason there are so many articles and books on diets and organization is because people don't change their behaviors and want an easier way to stay at their desired weight and/or organized without doing the work of changing behaviors.

Although patterns of behavior are difficult to change, they can be changed with effort. Making changes can be less difficult, and even fun, when done with other people who have a sense of humor.

You can find local communication groups or you can start one. This might even be a way to meet like-minded people while improving your communication skills!

How to Change Habits

There are many articles written on changing habits. They usually come out in the second week of February when the New Year's resolutions are forgotten, but we become concerned about issues of healthy habits for avoiding the winter blues, spring clothes that reveal more of our bodies, and organizing our papers for taxes. Here are some suggestions on changing communication habits that we have found useful:

- Don't try to change all your communication habits at once. Keep your goals achievable. Start by selecting one that you want to change.

- Realize that you are capable of learning this new action.

- Motivate yourself by what you will gain by making the change, such as avoiding conflicts created by misunderstandings or saving time through more effective and efficient communication.

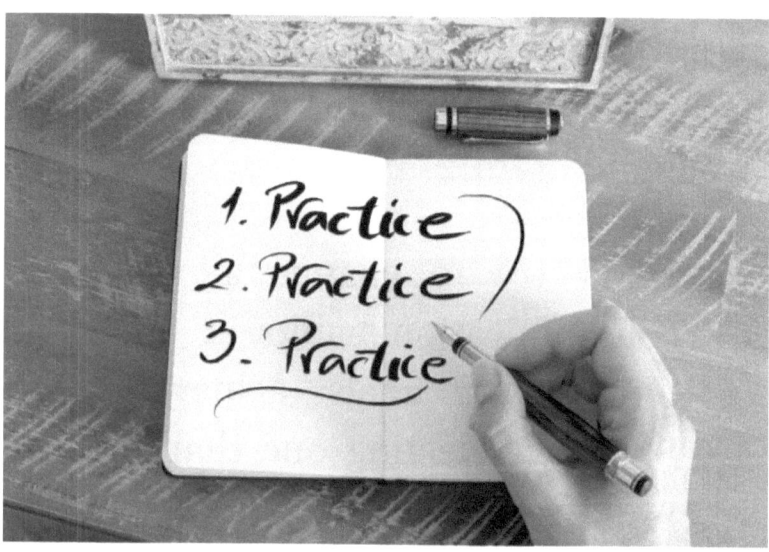

- On occasion, you might slip back into your old habit, but you will quickly correct it.

- Beware of triggers that might interfere with your good efforts! Sometimes it takes two to cooperate in order to solve communication challenges. Your communication partner has habits, too.

- Pause to think of your new habit every time before you start communicating. (This new action will take time in the beginning and you might think, "I don't have time for this!" Eventually, it will save you a lot of time because you will not have to repeat and clarify so often. When your new habit becomes automatic, you won't even have to think about it.)

- Take a moment each time you are successful with your new habit to congratulate yourself!

Personalize strategies for you

Working with your partner requires their effort. Perhaps the person with hearing loss calls you from the other room and expects to hear your answer? You know that they will not be able to understand you through the wall. Do you feel compelled to go to them each time? Problems like this need to be worked out in order to avoid conflicts and there are different ways of dealing with them.

A creative strategy worked for one couple: A woman complained that her husband with a hearing loss talked to her when she was in another part of the house, and he could never hear her answer. He kept saying "What? What?" until she went to him while he kept sitting in his easy chair!

She problem-solved and found a good time to tell him of the problem. He tried to change his habit, but he kept slipping back into talking to her from the other room. She was frustrated but determined to find a solution.

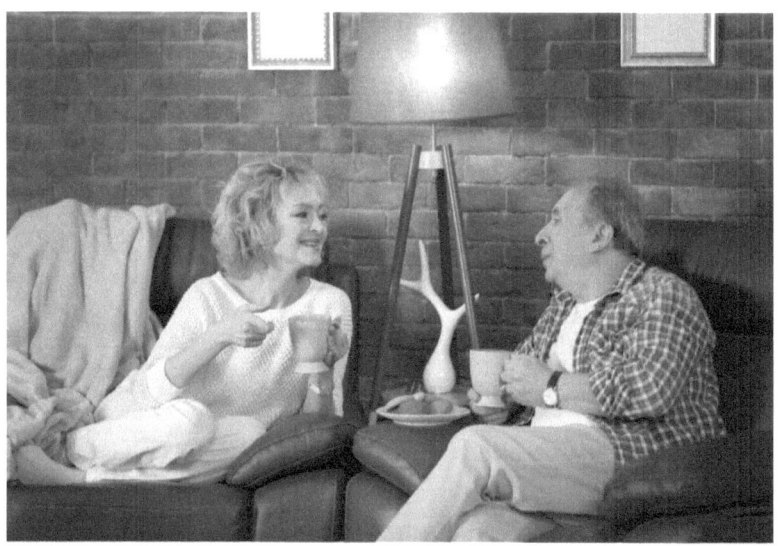

She told him that she would have the same reply whenever this happened to remind him. Every time he called her from another room, she sang loudly: "I can hear you, but I'm not coming!" and then waited. Although he could not understand all the words, he could hear her melody and he got the message! Either he got up from his chair and went to her, or he wrote it down so that he would not forget to tell her.

Clever ways to avoid conflicts can save marriages. Effective communication requires the cooperation of both partners and starts with understanding the problem.

Conclusion

Now that you understand more about living with hearing loss, we hope that you can communicate more effectively. Learning new habits can be difficult, so don't get discouraged. We all make mistakes. Keep practicing!

We always like to learn from the experiences of our readers. If you have comments and/or suggestions that might improve the next edition, we'd love to hear from you! You can contact us at:

TalkToPeopleWithHearingLoss@gmail.com

Acknowledgements

The authors would like to express our appreciation to people who encouraged us to write this book and/or gave helpful comments on an earlier version of the manuscript. They are:

Alison Cannon

Ann Hussey Hogaboom

Barbara Letts

Charles Kerr

Cynthia Healer

Fielding Brown

Joseph Dillion

Linda Mazie

Linda Welsh

Lisa Devlin

Lynn Hansberry Mayo

Marie Morgan

Mary M. Florentine

Michael Granat

Judy Potts   Nancy P. Hansberry

Karen Niglio   Richard A. Hogaboom

Kathy Granat   Richard Brown

Lawrence J. Epstein   Trine Ross

We are also grateful for the support of the Communication Focus Group at the Senior Center in Norwood, Massachusetts, including James Schmidt, Marsha Trementozzi, Joan McDermott, Helen "Bonnie" Bonaveto, and Executive Director Kerri McCarthy.

84

Further Resources

More information on ways to improve communication is readily available on a number of websites. There is also lots of other information and support for people with hearing loss, their friends, and families. We recommend the following resources, which cover:

- General information about hearing loss

- Advice for friends and family of people with hearing loss

- Support for people with hearing loss

- Other services worldwide

We have tried to organize the services under these categories, but many of them cover a mix of these areas and more. While some of them are national organizations, they offer useful information no matter where you are from!

General Information

World Health Organization (WHO) Fact Sheet

WHO is an international organization that works to promote health. This page is their Deafness and Hearing Loss Fact Sheet, which has information about hearing loss statistics, causes, impacts, prevention, identification, and management.

who.int/en/news-room/fact-sheets/detail/deafness-and-hearing-loss

Mayo Clinic

The Mayo Clinic is a nonprofit organization that treats and researches a wide range of conditions. This page has information about the symptoms and causes of hearing loss. It also does a good job of explaining the difference between conductive and sensorineural hearing loss.

mayoclinic.org/diseases-conditions/hearing-loss/symptoms-causes/syc-20373072

National Institute on Deafness and other Communication Disorders (NIDCD)

Part of the National Institutes of Health (NIH), which is the American government's focal point for biomedical research, NIDCD supports research and training related to disease prevention and health promotion. The information on this page is mainly for people with hearing loss, but also describes what friends and family can do to help.

nidcd.nih.gov/health/age-related-hearing-loss

National Institute on Aging (NIA)

NIA is an American organization, which is also part of NIH. It supports research and education for older people. This page includes general information about hearing loss and how to talk to people with hearing loss.

nia.nih.gov/health/hearing-loss-common-problem-older-adults

Centers for Disease Control and Prevention (CDC)

The CDC is an American government organization that works to prevent disease. They have three pages with information about hearing loss in children, resources for young adults, and preventing hearing loss caused by workplace noise.

cdc.gov/hearingloss

The Hearing Foundation of Canada

The Hearing Foundation of Canada is a national nonprofit that promotes prevention, research, and intervention. Their website has general information about hearing health and hearing loss. They also have stories about people with hearing loss and their families.

hearingfoundation.ca

Advice for Friends and Family

Hear-It AISBL

Hear-it is an international non-profit in Brussels (AISBL is a French acronym referring to non-profits in Belgium), which collects and distributes information about hearing loss. Their website has lots of information, and this page has resources for friends and family of people with hearing loss.

hear-it.org/somebody-close-has-hearing-loss

Action on Hearing Loss

Action on Hearing Loss (formerly RNID) is the UK's largest charity helping people with life-changing hearing loss, deafness, and tinnitus. They fund research, challenge stigma, run an information line, have online forums, and offer training, information, and advice. The page below provides information for friends and family of people with hearing loss, including how to approach them about the issue.

actiononhearingloss.org.uk/how-we-help/friends-and-family

MedlinePlus

Medline Plus is the NIH website for patients, family and friends, which gives information about diseases, conditions, and wellness in plain language. This page has some specific tips on how to talk to people with hearing loss.

medlineplus.gov/ency/patientinstruction s/000361.htm

Canadian Hard of Hearing Association (CHHA)

The CHHA is a nonprofit that aims to empower Canadians with hearing loss through education, public awareness, service, and advocacy. They have a range of information about hearing loss on their website, including the page below, which has tips on communicating with people with hearing loss.

chha.ca/hearing-education/living-with-hearing-loss/#Tips

Hearing Help

The Hearing Help website is an initiative of Australian Hearing, Australia's largest provider of government-funded hearing services. On their website you can call or live chat with a hearing specialist and find a range of self-help tools. This page has a range of articles for friends and family of people with hearing loss, including tips on how to find restaurants that are ideal for people with hearing loss!

hearinghelp.com.au/helping-others

Hearing Matters Australia

Hearing Matters Australia (formally Self-Help for Hard of Hearing) is a voluntary, non-profit, peer-support organization for people with hearing loss. Part of their mission is also to educate and support friends and family. They have many information pages, including this guide for people with hearing loss on how to improve their communication.

94

shhhaust.org/ideas-for-hearing-impaired-people-improving-communication

Hearing Loss Support

Hearing Loss Association of America (HLAA)

The HLAA is America's leading organization representing consumers with hearing loss. Their main purpose is to educate people about hearing loss, support people with hearing loss, and advocate for them. Their website has a wide range of resources, including basic hearing loss information, finding a professional, a guide to hearing loss technology, advocacy news, financial assistance, and events.

hearingloss.org

HEARnet

HEARnet is an Australian website that offers independent and easily understandable information about the types of hearing loss and the ways hearing loss can be managed.

hearnet.org.au

Hearing Link

This is a UK charity that is specifically for people with hearing loss. Their helpdesk offers free, confidential support and independent information. They offer free support groups (called LinkUps) for people with hearing loss and their friends/family. They also have community support volunteers, who visit people with hearing loss and their families to help manage hearing loss and get the best from services.

hearinglink.org

Cleveland Clinic

The Cleveland Clinic is a nonprofit academic medical center with a range of specialties. They offer medical care, research, and education. This page has a range of resources, including statistics, information about hearing aids, and a guide for treatment options for both adults and children.

my.clevelandclinic.org/departments/hea d-neck/patient-education/hearing-loss-resources

National Health Service (NHS)

The UK's national health service website offers information about hearing loss prevention and treatment.

nhs.uk/conditions/hearing-loss

Better Hearing Australia

Better Hearing Australia is an independent expert organization in hearing loss management. Their website has a number of information pages and they run a hearing advice helpline.

betterhearing.org.au

The SayWhatClub

The SayWhatClub is an international nonprofit peer-to-peer support organization run by volunteers with hearing loss. They have a Facebook group and an email mailing list.

saywhatclub.org

Other Services Worldwide

More support in other countries and other international organizations can be found here:

hear-it.org/organisations-for-hearing-impaired-people

www.ingramcontent.com/pod-product-compliance
Lightning Source LLC
Chambersburg PA
CBHW030403290526
45785CB00004B/1882